The Complete Guide to ACL Rehab

How to heal your anterior cruciate ligament after injury

Natty Bandasak

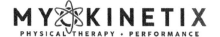

The Complete Guide to ACL Rehab:
How to heal your anterior cruciate ligament after injury
by Natty Bandasak

Published by Myokinetix
Englewood, NJ
United States of America

Book design and formatting by
Leesa Ellis of 3 ferns books >> **www.3fernsbooks.com**

Library of Congress Control Number: 2022901942

ISBN (paperback): 979-8-9854720-0-4
ISBN (hardback): 979-8-9854720-2-8
ISBN (e-book): 979-8-9854720-1-1

Table of Contents

Chapter 1

Foreword

Introducing Dr. Natty Bandasak, PT, DPT, Founder of Myokinetix Physical Therapy and Performance:

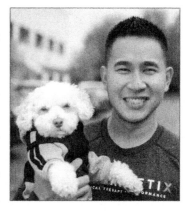

ACL tears are one of the hardest injuries to overcome. They require both immense physical and mental strength to endure the 10-12 months of rehabilitation. But being able to guide my patients through their journey is incredibly rewarding, especially once they see that they can get back on the field - stronger, faster, more flexible, and with greater confidence in themselves.

Since the start of my career, my goals have centered on putting the patient first. But I found myself stuck in a toxic clinic environment that rewarded high patient volume and enabled low standards when it came to receiving quality care. For me, this was the pivotal moment when I realized that something had to give.

Overworked and burned out, I dreamt of creating a world class environment where amateur athletes, professionals, and weekend warriors alike could train like VIPs. From this inspiration, Myokinetix Physical Therapy and Performance was born.

At Myokinetix Physical Therapy and Performance, you'll never have to worry about being just a number. We pride ourselves in the "People over Profit" mentality and take the time to truly understand your goals and limitations. As experts in treating ACL injuries, our goal is to share knowledge on the most up-to-date research about ACL injuries and the recovery process with athletes, parents, and coaches. This book will achieve this goal by sharing the evidence-based information, a recovery road map, Do's and Don'ts, and exercises that are necessary to get back on the field.

What To Expect
In This Book

This book is a compilation of my knowledge and experiences from years of treating ACL injuries. I have included the most important information for your recovery here; however, before starting or trying any sort of exercise program, always consult with a physical therapist first.

Where To Find More Information

This book is accompanied by a catalog of exercises, as well as some additional information, which you can find by scanning the QR code below.

Chapter 2

About the ACL and ACL Injuries

ACL tears are some of the most recognized injuries in sports and athletics. Many are aware of the devastating consequences that come from ACL injuries, ranging from surgery to missed games. Add to that several months of rehabilitation and recovery, and it's easy to see why these athletes with ACL tears miss entire seasons of competition.

But why does ACL recovery take so long? To answer this question and more, it's important to learn the basics about the ACL and contributing factors to the injury itself.

About the ACL

The Anterior Cruciate Ligament (ACL) is found inside the knee joint and connects the femur to the tibia. Although it's incredibly strong, the ligament itself has very little elasticity. As a result, it absorbs large amounts of stress until it stretches or weakens, and then it tears.

An ACL tear usually occurs as a result of:

* Cutting or pivoting maneuvers, like when an athlete plants a foot and suddenly shifts direction

* Landing on one leg

* When the knee is hit directly, especially when it is hyper-extended or bent inward

* Deceleration from running

* Repeated stress to the knee

* Falling on a bent or twisted knee

Signs of an ACL Injury

It's important to realize that, while some signs and symptoms occur immediately after injury to the ACL, others may appear or worsen over the next few days.

Some of the most common signs and symptoms of an ACL injury are:

* Sudden, sharp pain

* Immediate swelling and warmth in the knee joint

* Deep, aching pain in the joint that worsens with walking or climbing stairs

* Feeling as if the knee is "giving out"

* Limited range of motion

* Tenderness and bruising around the area

Lesser Known Facts About ACL Injury

It is believed that more than 200,000 cases of ACL injuries occur each year. However, exact estimates are hard to come by since there is no standard method to track the number of ACL tears in a given year.

The ACL is the most commonly injured structure in the knee, accounting for more than 50% of all knee injuries.

A majority, about 60–70%, of ACL tears occur by non-contact, meaning there is no collision with another person or object. Surprisingly, research has found that athletes who ski or play soccer and basketball are at the highest risk for a non-contact ACL tear. Conversely, those who play football are most vulnerable to an ACL tear due to direct contact.

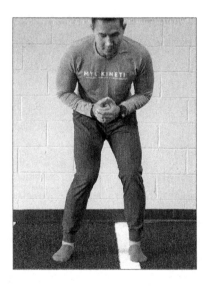 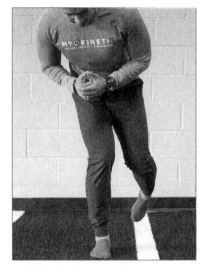

ACL Injuries in Males

Males and females both share the same mechanism of ACL injury, which is typically a rapid but awkward stop and anticipation of lateral movements. However, males are statistically less likely to have an ACL injury than females, as has been seen in a variety of data that has been collected.

ACL Injuries in Females

Females are more prone to ACL injuries than males. This fact has been echoed by many experts, most notably by Myer and colleagues in an article published by the *Strength and Conditioning Journal*.[1]

According to this article published in the *Journal of Orthopaedics*, the incidence of female ACL injury is 3.5 times that of male injury in basketball and 2.8 times that of male injury in soccer.[2]

There are a number of reasons why women may have an increased risk of ACL injury. Due to structural differences between male and female bodies, women may have more stress on the soft tissues surrounding the knee joint. One difference that is commonly seen in women is known as knee valgus, which refers to the angle between the knee joint. Knee valgus places more stress on the ACL, thus increasing the risk for an ACL tear.

Additionally, due to the common size difference between females and males, women tend to have less muscle surrounding the knee joint. This, combined with the fact that female bodies tend to rely more upon the quadriceps, which are significantly less effective than the hamstrings at controlling the knee joint, during deceleration, places huge amounts of stress on the ACL that can lead to instability and a higher chance of a tear if it is overstretched.

---

1   Nyman, E., Jr, & Armstrong, C. W. (2015). Real-time feedback during drop landing training improves subsequent frontal and sagittal plane knee kinematics. *Clinical biomechanics (Bristol, Avon), 30*(9), 988–994.

2   The female ACL: Why is it more prone to injury?. (2016). *Journal of orthopaedics, 13*(2), A1–A4.

Finally, some experts think that hormone levels may play a part in the different injury rates between women and men. Women have less testosterone and more estrogen than men, which may contribute to increased looseness in tendons and ligaments, another area of concern when it comes to ACL injury.

ACL Injuries in Children and Teens

A major cause for concern when it comes to ACL injury in children and teens is specializing in one sport at a young age. According to several studies, an emphasis on playing one sport, known as sport specialization, leads to overuse injuries, overtraining, and mental burnout. Sports specialization is defined as participating in one sport for more than eight months of the year, participation in one sport to the point that others are excluded, and sports that involve those younger than 12 years old.

The American Orthopedic Society for Sports Medicine strongly opposes early sport specialization for several reasons. Their consensus statement cites long-term physical and mental dangers, such as sleep dysfunction, eating disorders, isolation from peers, higher levels of stress and anxiety, and ineffective coping strategies, and presents data to suggest that those who play multiple sports are more likely to play professionally than those who limit themselves to one sport.[3]

Parents of young children should also keep in mind that a lack of expertise and guidance when it comes to physical conditioning is a significant risk factor for sports injuries. Without proper guidance to develop motor skills, children are predisposed to poor movement patterns that alter their ability to run, jump, or turn and in turn increase the risk for ACL injury.

---

3   LaPrade, R. F., Agel, J., Baker, J., Brenner, J. S., Cordasco, F. A., Côté, J., Engebretsen, L., Feeley, B. T., Gould, D., Hainline, B., Hewett, T. E., Jayanthi, N., Kocher, M. S., Myer, G. D., Nissen, C. W., Philippon, M. J., & Provencher, M. T. (2016). AOSSM Early Sport Specialization Consensus Statement. *Orthopaedic Journal of Sports Medicine*.

Contributing Risk Factors to an ACL Knee Injury

A delicate balance between your muscles, bones, and ligaments allows your body to move freely without restriction or pain. When muscles are weak or injured, the ligaments and tendons are forced to do more work to support your bones. Over time, the ligaments become overstretched, overstressed, and weak. This, combined with specific sport maneuvers, creates the perfect storm for an ACL tear.

There are two categories of factors that can predispose you to an ACL injury: modifiable and non-modifiable factors. Non-modifiable factors cannot be changed to lessen your risk of injury, and include things like genetics, gender, a previous history of ACL injury, and the size of your ACL ligament.

The second category is referred to as modifiable factors, which means they can be changed or altered in some way. Modifiable factors that might affect one's risk for an ACL tear include:

Body mass index

Experts believe that having a higher body mass index (BMI) predisposes one to ACL tears and arthritis, especially in men and non-contact ACL injuries. There's also evidence that points to people with higher BMI having weaker muscles surrounding the knee joint, which increases the risk for injury.

Playing surface

Research on the controversy regarding artificial turf versus grass is divided. According to years of data gathered by the National Collegiate Athletic Association on collegiate soccer players, athletes are 8.7x more likely to sustain an ACL injury during practice on natural grass compared with practice on artificial turf.[4] However,

4   Howard, M., Solaru, S., Kang, H. P., Bolia, I. K., Hatch, G., Tibone, J. E., Gamradt, S. C., & Weber, A. E. (2020). Epidemiology of Anterior Cruciate Ligament Injury on Natural Grass Versus Artificial Turf in Soccer: 10-Year Data From the National Collegiate Athletic Association Injury Surveillance System. *Orthopaedic journal of sports medicine, 8*(7).

it's important to realize that the overall risk of injury is small, regardless of gender. Interestingly, another study published in 2019 on collegiate football found that the risk of ACL injuries in those who competed in lower divisions (Division II and III) was higher on artificial turf than on grass.

Jumping mechanics technique

Knee valgus, a medical term that describes abnormal inward positioning of the knee, is a recognized risk factor for lower body injuries, especially ACL tears. When the knee collapses inward during movement, like jumping, it is known as a dynamic knee valgus that causes abnormal positioning at the hip, knee, and ankle. Additionally, valgus is one of the foremost risk factors for acute (new) and chronic injuries due to its catastrophic effects on your bones, muscles, ligaments, and tendons. Those with large muscle imbalances between the quad muscles (strong) and hamstrings (weaker), poor balance, and decreased core control/ability are at risk for developing knee valgus.

Although knee valgus can be influenced by genetics and bone structure, there are strategies to prevent it from worsening or leading to injury. These include retraining movement patterns, hip strengthening, proprioceptive/balance exercises, and agility training.

Having one, or more than one, risk factor does not necessarily mean that you'll suffer an ACL injury. However, it does increase the probability, especially if you play a sport that requires frequent and sudden *deceleration or cutting, pivoting, and jumping on one leg.*

The aforementioned modifiable factors are often discussed when it comes to ACL knee injuries, but we want to talk about others you may not be aware of. For example, did you know that mental fatigue can raise your risk of sustaining an ACL tear? Mental fatigue can result from bad sleep habits, lack of recovery time between games, or incomplete physical recovery. It plays a major role in your ability to concentrate, focus, and pay attention which are obvious risk factors for any injury.

Chapter 3

Surgery for an ACL Tear

The number one question after sustaining an ACL tear is, "Will I need surgery?" And truth be told, about 77% of ACL injuries will.

Surgery for an ACL tear involves reconstructing the torn ligament using something called a graft. Reconstructions are necessary because, oftentimes, the torn fragments of the ACL are beyond repair. The surgeon reconstructs your ACL using a graft from a different tendon in the body (autograft) or a donor graft from another source (allograft).

The material in the graft acts as the foundation for the new ligament to grow on. Below are the most common autografts used in surgery for an ACL tear.

* **Patellar tendon.** Your patellar tendon is used to replace the torn ACL. Recovery is usually uncomplicated, and its strength makes the patellar tendon a popular choice for elite athletes.

* **Hamstring tendon.** Becoming more common, hamstring tendon autographs have been shown to decrease knee pain and recovery time compared to patellar tendon grafts.

* **Quadriceps tendon.** Quadriceps tendon autografts are often used for ACL revision surgery.

The graft selection is determined by your surgeon. However, you should know that no specific graft type has been proven to be superior to the others.

What to Expect During and After ACL Surgery

Initially, ACL surgery will make your knee feel weak and unstable. This is caused by pain and swelling related to the surgery. You'll follow up with your surgeon a few days later to have your incision and bandages checked.

Specific precautions and instructions will be made by your surgeon, and it's imperative that you follow them for the best outcomes after ACL surgery. Most surgeons will protect the knee in a brace that extends from your ankle to your thigh. For the first few days, your brace is locked in extension, meaning you won't be able to bend the leg. As your strength and knee control improve, your brace will be unlocked to allow for more movement. The brace can be removed for showering and exercising unless otherwise directed by your surgeon.

It's likely that you'll leave the hospital with crutches to help you move around for the first few weeks. Depending on your specific graft, your surgeon may give you specific instructions for weight-bearing on your affected side. You can expect weight-bearing precautions ranging from 50–100%, followed by full weight-bearing by the end of the second week after surgery.

Recovery

GENERAL STATISTICS

Pain medication is generally recommended after ACL surgery and during the first phase of rehabilitation to decrease pain from the surgical procedure. It plays an important role, especially during physical therapy, when it helps override the brain's automatic pain response to protect the knee and increase tension in the surrounding muscles. This can cause difficulties in bending and straightening the knee. But pain medication can help decrease pain levels and allow for a greater range of motion to be achieved during physical therapy sessions.

POSSIBILITY OF REINJURY

Despite the generally positive outlook for ACL surgeries, there is a well-documented chance of reinjury, which is higher in both females and children.[5]

Statistics vary according to the source, but recent literature suggests that one in five young athletes will suffer from another ACL injury at some point in their career.[6] Additionally, the rate of reinjury in those who return to play is about 40x greater than athletes without a history of ACL injury. Most recently, the *Journal of Orthopaedic & Sports Physical Therapy* published shocking results that showed athletes returning to sports after ACL surgery prior to nine months are 7x more likely to sustain a second ACL injury, even up to two years later.[7]

---

5   Barber-Westin, S., & Noyes, F. R. (2020). One in 5 Athletes Sustain Reinjury Upon Return to High-Risk Sports After ACL Reconstruction: A Systematic Review in 1239 Athletes Younger Than 20 Years. *Sports health, 12*(6), 587–597.
6   Ibid.
7   Beischer, S., Gustavsson, L., Senorski, E. H., Karlsson, J., Thomeé, C., Samuelsson, K., & Thomeé, R. (2020). Young Athletes Who Return to Sport Before 9 Months After Anterior Cruciate Ligament Reconstruction Have a Rate of New Injury 7 Times That of Those Who Delay Return. *The Journal of orthopaedic and sports physical therapy, 50*(2), 83–90.

Tips to Ensure the Best Outcome After ACL Surgery

You may be surprised to hear that most people can move the knee immediately after surgery for an ACL tear. Rehabilitation begins shortly thereafter in order to achieve these goals:

* Improve range of motion

* Increase strength

* Decrease swelling

* Reintroduce walking

* Restore balance and proprioception

Some surgeons may recommend the use of knee braces; however, there is no evidence to link them with decreased recovery time or better outcomes.

Achieving specific goals after surgery may make the difference between a full and incomplete recovery from an ACL tear. Regaining full motion, especially leg extension, on both sides of the body is critical for recovery and will affect future episodes of knee pain. Research has found that the critical window for regaining that full leg extension is within the *first two weeks after ACL surgery.*

But there are plenty of other factors to consider when it comes to rehabilitating a newly repaired ACL. You may not know this, but sleep, nutrition, hydration, and behavioral health should all be entered into the recovery plan.

Let's explore these factors more closely to learn the things you should be doing during recovery from an ACL tear.

Get plenty of sleep after ACL surgery.

The biggest sleep-related concern with a repaired ACL is a lack of sleep. In this wheelhouse, goals for recovery include quality sleep, decreasing pain levels, and limiting heavy pain medication use.

Think about it – surgery (and recovery) is painful. Afterward, you may have problems falling asleep and/or be getting less sleep than usual. This becomes problematic because the less you sleep, the more sensitive you are to that pain. Aside from obvious fatigue, this can lead to increased use of opioids prescribed after surgery.

There are a couple of ways to combat sleep deprivation. Sleep aids can be effective in decreasing the amount of time it takes to fall asleep at night as well as increasing time asleep. Unfortunately, a medicated sleep aid does not have the same health benefits as normal sleep does. So even though it may help you fall (and stay) asleep at night after an ACL repair, it does not benefit you as much as Cognitive Behavioral Therapy.

Cognitive Behavioral Therapy (CBT) is a form of therapy that focuses on changing thoughts and behaviors to manage pain. And it's pretty effective in doing so – which means less pain and more sleep.

People notice these effects after trying CBT:

✱ Improved their sleep efficiency

✱ Fewer interruptions during the night

✱ Quicker to fall asleep

✱ Improved quality of sleep

Case in point: making sleep a priority during your ACL rehabilitation will foster a quick recovery. But what happens when you're struggling to get restful sleep and desperate to find a solution? Try mindfulness meditation and guided breathing exercises, such as body scan technique. Both are designed to increase your awareness in the moment to theoretically reduce fears and calm anxious thoughts about the past or future.

Mindfulness meditation is the practice of sharpening your awareness the exact moment you are in. It also teaches you how to pay attention to the present moment with openness and acceptance, making mindfulness meditation a popular practice with those who suffer from chronic pain. Current research shows that it can reduce symptoms of pain, improve your mood, reduce feelings of anxiety and depression, and may decrease your need for pain medication.[8] Mindfulness does this by encouraging you to focus on your breathing rhythm. When we are mindful of ourselves, we pay more attention to what we are doing while worrying less about other things. As you can see, it's the opposite of going through the motions since you are tuned into your senses, body, thoughts, and emotions. To practice mindfulness meditation, find a quiet place where you won't be disturbed. Follow your breath and bring your attention to the physical sensations of breathing through your nose, chest, or mouth. Practice observing your thoughts, wherever they may go, and gently guide them back without judgment or expectation.

Guided breathing exercises, like the body scan technique, are useful to bring awareness to the body, especially during times of injury. By mentally scanning yourself from head to toe, you can assess the relationship between your mind and body to improve your sleep, reduce stress, and hone your focus. To do the body scan

8   Hilton, L., Hempel, S., Ewing, B. A., Apaydin, E., Xenakis, L., Newberry, S., Colaiaco, B., Maher, A. R., Shanman, R. M., Sorbero, M. E., & Maglione, M. A. (2017). Mindfulness Meditation for Chronic Pain: Systematic Review and Meta-analysis. *Annals of behavioral medicine : a publication of the Society of Behavioral Medicine, 51*(2), 199–213.

technique, close your eyes as you draw your attention to your head and neck. Check for feelings, sensations, or pain for 30 seconds before moving down to the shoulders and upper back. Repeat for your arms, hands, chest, low back, stomach, hips, legs, and feet. Avoid the temptation to try to change the sensation that you're noticing and, instead, simply notice it, and breathe through it.

Prioritize nutrition and good eating habits during ACL recovery.

With an ACL injury or surgery, you're bound to have a good deal of inflammation/swelling and pain. Fortunately, nutrition is a great way to combat inflammation from the inside out.[9]

In addition to controlling inflammation, upping your nutrition game can play a key role in providing the nutrients that your body needs to rebuild itself and reducing the risk of muscle loss. And, according to experts, surgery can require 20% more calories than being at rest.[10] After surgery, it's recommended that you increase your fluid and fiber intake to reduce feelings of constipation that is a common side effect of the procedure and pain medication.

There are a handful of anti-inflammatory foods and supplements that can be beneficial to the recovery process. But when it comes to nutrition, it's important to acknowledge that these needs are going to vary case-by-case.

What do we mean by this? Let's take a look.

---

9   Knappenberger, K., MS, RD, CSSD, ATC. Nutrition for Injury Recovery and Rehabilitation. National Athletic Trainers' Association. https://www.nata. org/sites/default/files/nutrition-for-injury-recovery-and-rehabilitation.pdf

10 Tipton K. D. (2015). Nutritional Support for Exercise-Induced Injuries. *Sports medicine (Auckland, N.Z.), 45* Suppl 1, S93–S104.

Omega-3 fats are effective in reducing muscle loss and preventing inflammation. You can find them in the following foods:

* Nuts or nut butter

* Seeds

* Avocado

* Oily fish

* Flaxseed oil

* Extra Virgin Olive Oil (EVOO)

* Omega-3 fish oil

Proteins will help with muscle growth and recovery as you heal from ACL surgery. Add nuts and seeds, beans, cod, tuna, chicken, and steak to meet your needs in this category – they'll provide you with the protein you need and help combat inflammation along the way.

Fiber is beneficial in reducing constipation, a common side effect of the pain medication that comes with an ACL repair. This can be found in prunes or prune juice, whole grains, and various fruits and vegetables.

Vitamins and minerals can be used either supplementally or within your diet. The following can provide a wide range of benefits during the recovery process of an ACL tear:

* **Vitamin A aids in cell growth and development.**
  Incorporate this into your diet with sweet potatoes, spinach, and carrots.

* **Vitamin C can help with wound healing and tissue repair.**
  You can find it in broccoli and citrus fruits.

* **Vitamin D is a big player in bone health and immune function.**
  Look for salmon, tuna, and mushrooms to add Vitamin D to your diet.

* **Calcium is a key mineral for skeletal structure and function – aka, keeping your bones in good shape.**
  Broccoli, seeds, and dairy products (of course) will provide your diet with a calcium boost.

* **Copper comes into play with red blood cell formation, immune function, and bone health.**
  It is found in nuts and seeds, leafy greens, and lobster.

* **Zinc is effective in aiding wound healing, protein synthesis, and immune function.**
  Between meat, shellfish, and legumes, there's plenty of ways to add zinc to your diet.

There are a few other supplemental nutrients that benefit the recovery process. Tart cherry juice and fish oil can fight inflammation, and casein proteins prevent muscle breakdown. Branch chain amino acids (also known as BCAAs) are useful to strengthen muscles, tendons, and ligaments. Collagen helps boost muscle mass and relieve joint pain.

While these are great additions to your diet, there are also things you should avoid. Not to state the obvious, but nutrient deficiencies won't get you very far when it comes to recovery. Omega-6 fats, such as vegetable oil and saturated fats, actually increase inflammation and should be avoided. Added sugar in the diet is a no-go too, as it will also increase inflammation.

Staying hydrated helps you to recover after ACL surgery.

To keep it short and sweet, hydration is incredibly important to ACL recovery.

Athletes typically maintain good hydration levels because they are so active – and an ACL injury should not be any different. In fact, the best practice is to drink as much water as you normally would.

The body is made up of 60% water. That's more than half of our body composition, and it cannot afford to be compromised when it comes to ACL recovery. Water is effective[11] in flushing toxins out of our system, especially anesthesia after surgery, and aiding in the anti-inflammatory response.[12]

Try to drink between ¾ gallon to a full gallon of water per day. If water is too bland for you, try flavored water – but be careful of those added sugars. Feel free to incorporate fruits into your diet since they can offer little spurts of hydration and provide a break in the routine.

Don't neglect your mental health during your ACL recovery.

An ACL tear can be particularly devastating to an athlete. Most athletes look at an ACL injury as the end all be all – the season-ending knee injury that you never fully come back from. However, with a little bit of encouragement, recovery outcomes are positive.

Now would be a good time to do a thorough social media audit and cleansing. Channel your inner Marie Kondo by unfollowing pages and influencers who do not bring you joy, lift your spirit, and bring you encouragement. Instead, find pages, groups, or informative podcasts, like the Myokinetix Podcast, related to ACL injury and recovery to keep you on the right path with a positive mindset.

---

11   Kehlet H. (2020). Enhanced postoperative recovery: good from afar, but far from good?. *Anaesthesia, 75 Suppl 1*, e54–e61.

12   Gupta, R. and Gan, T.J. (2016), Peri-operative fluid management to enhance recovery. *Anaesthesia, 71:* 40-45.

Now, let's touch upon why this is so important.

Most commonly, athletes struggle with hesitation and lack of confidence in the recovery process. This is a self-limiting behavior to avoid reinjury. You may be exhibiting low confidence behaviors if you find yourself:

* Decreasing the intensity of your activity

* Relying on a knee brace

* Perceiving your knee as unstable

Coming to terms with an ACL injury is something athletes tend to struggle with as well. As said before, they see it as season-ending. Some even begin to assume that their entire athletic career is over. Oftentimes, this negative thought process leads to questions about their future athletic career.

Though an ACL tear is not a career-ending injury, there is a decision to be made. Athletes who return to sport will face the possibility of a repeat injury. Recovery offers time for reflection and re-prioritization. For most, there is a lot more to life than being an athlete. Depending on when the injury occurred in your career, you may have life plans that a 10 month recovery time doesn't fit into. You have the option to make the call on "hanging up your cleats" at any point during the recovery process.

Expectations and assumptions about the rehabilitation and recovery process are other limiting factors to recovery from ACL surgery. Admittedly, long physical therapy sessions can be frustrating and appear to be never-ending. It can feel like you're going nowhere fast, and that's discouraging. Along with that, the inability to complete basic tasks (especially right after surgery) can be a big knock to the ego.

But rest assured, the most important thing to know when rehabilitating an ACL injury is that, even though it may take a while, the outcomes are good. Here are a few tips that are proven to help your mindset as you recover from an ACL injury:

* **You need a strong support system.** Surrounding yourself with people who cheer you on and help cope with recovery can increase your confidence in the process.

* Self-efficacy is the belief that you can perform a task successfully. **Believing in your ability** to attain your goals plays a major role in positive rehabilitation outcomes.

* **Continue to participate in team activities.** Remaining with your team while you recover is a great way to motivate yourself. Do your rehab exercises at practice and participate in team activities. Seeing your teammates on the field can encourage you to want to be back out there with them.

* **Setting short-term goals** is a great way to make the recovery process fly by. Long-term goals can be frustrating, but individualized short-term goals are motivating when it comes to returning to play.

* **Incorporate meditation into your rehabilitation.** Meditation is a fantastic way to increase mindfulness, which helps you reach a more relaxed state of mind. It can come in the form of something as simple as lying still and controlling your breathing or something more active, such as a walking meditation. This can lead to lower anxiety levels and increased outcomes during your recovery.

* **Visualize your recovery** by utilizing mental imagery. Mentally rehearse the different exercises for your rehabilitation and visualize what your knee looks like as it recovers from an ACL injury. This can reduce your stress - known to have a negative effect on the healing process.

* **Celebrate your goals**. Every small win is a win, and each one should be celebrated. Getting excited about how far you've come will play a huge role in the confidence department.

Chapter 4

Phase I Rehab after ACL Surgery

Once you decide to have surgery for an ACL injury, you're likely to have many questions related to the recovery time, the rehab process, or when you'll be able to return to your normal routine.

First of all, it's crucial that you discuss any and all questions about your upcoming ACL surgery with your surgeon and medical team. They will be able to share detailed information about the procedure, your anticipated recovery time, and any special precautions that you'll need to take after surgery. These conversations will help you mentally prepare for the recovery ahead.

Rehab begins the day after your ACL surgery. While surgery for an ACL tear doesn't take very long (about 1-2 hours), it is still considered to be major surgery. Make arrangements with your school or employer to take some time off, especially right after surgery. Ask family or friends to help you with meals, household duties, and transportation to rehab since you won't be able to drive.

Controlling Pain and Swelling Early After ACL Surgery

For the first few days after ACL surgery, you may notice drainage and blood on your knee bandages. This is normal and necessary to avoid excessive swelling in the joint. You should monitor your bandages and be sure to keep the incisions dry until your stitches are removed.

Swelling after ACL surgery is managed by following these instructions:

* Avoid sitting with your leg down on the floor. Instead, elevate it on several pillows.

* Apply ice 4-5 times per day for 20 minutes. Your surgeon will have further Instructions regarding cold therapy.

* Perform ankle pumps to lower the risk for blood clots and swelling in the ankle and foot.

* Refrain from overdoing it for the first few days. Rest, ice, and elevate your leg as much as possible.

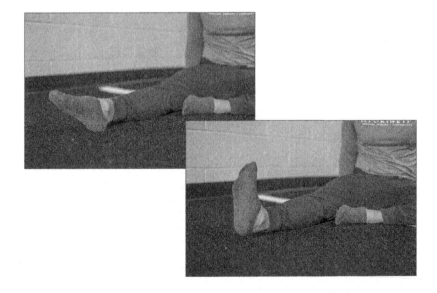

Recommendations for pain control will vary from surgeon to surgeon. You may be sent home with prescriptions for narcotics, anti-inflammatory medications, or nonsteroidal anti-inflammatory medications. Be sure to follow all instructions as directed on the prescription labels.

Chapter 5

Phase I Rehab

Phase I of ACL recovery and rehab begins immediately following surgery and lasts up to two weeks. During this phase, you will see your physical therapist about once or twice a week.

The main goals for Phase I are to *protect the knee, encourage healing, regain full knee extension (straightening), and be able to bend the knee to 90 degrees.* These goals are accomplished by controlling swelling and pain, taking care of the bandages, and introducing easy range of motion exercises.

You may be wondering why range of motion is encouraged before knee strengthening. This is because the most common complication after ACL surgery is loss of motion, especially knee extension. Loss of knee extension can cause a limp while walking, weak quads, and knee pain. Therefore, all early ACL recovery protocols focus on regaining range of motion as soon as possible.

This book is accompanied by a catalog of exercises, as well as some additional information, which you can find by scanning the QR code below.

Phase I ACL Exercises

All exercises should be relatively pain-free. Additionally, your physical therapist will perform something called patellar mobilizations, which is a fancy term for making sure your kneecap can move well.

Knee extension stretch

* Position the heel on a pillow or rolled towel with the knee unsupported. Make sure the heel is positioned high enough to lift the thigh off the table.

* Stay in this position for 10 to 15 minutes.

Heel slides with towel

* Lie on your back and place a towel underneath the heel of the operated knee.

* Slowly pull the heel toward your body, bending the knee. Once you feel a comfortable stretch, hold for 5 seconds.

* Straighten the leg by sliding the heel downward. Hold for 5 seconds and repeat.

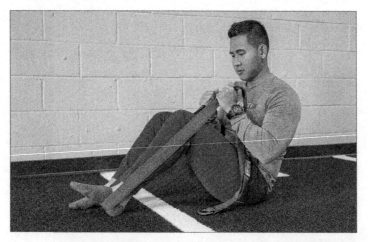

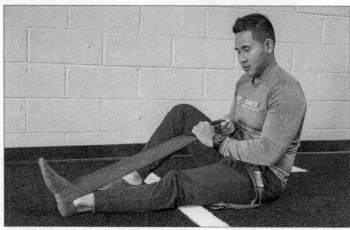

Figure 1: Heel slide.

Isometric quad contraction

* Straighten the operated leg in front of you.

* Press the knee down towards the ground. Hold for 5 seconds and then relax.

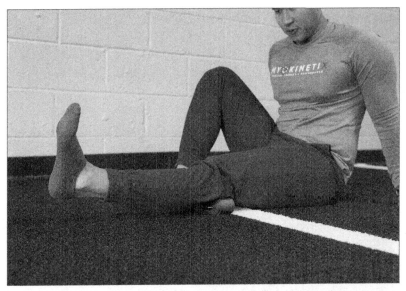

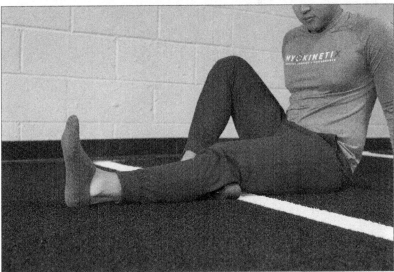

Figure 2: Quads set.

Straight leg raise with the knee brace

✱ Lie on your back and bend the unoperated knee. Straighten the operated leg and make sure the knee brace is locked in extension.

✱ Performing an isometric quad contraction with the leg to "lock" the knee and prevent excessive stress on the healing ACL graft.

✱ Gently lift the leg to about 45–60 degrees. Hold for 5 seconds.

✱ Slowly lower the leg back to the starting position. Relax the muscles.

✱ Once you can hold the quad contraction without allowing the leg to bend, known as a quad lag, then you can do this exercise without the knee brace.

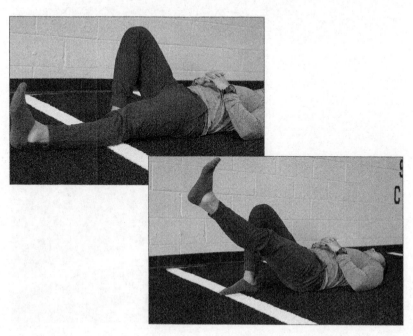

Figure 3: Straight leg raise.

Weight shifting exercises

✷ Stand behind a countertop or table and place both hands firmly on the surface. Position your feet about hip-width apart. Keep your knee brace on.

✷ Practice slowly shifting your weight from side to side. This helps your operated leg to regain stability and control at the knee joint.

✷ Hold each weight shift for 5 seconds.

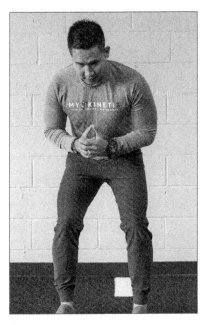 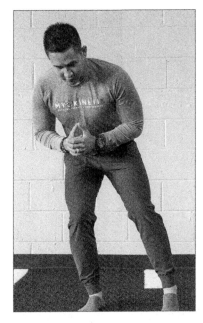

Figure 4: Weight-shifting.

By the end of the first week, you should have regained the ability to fully straighten the knee, bend at least 90 degrees, and regain some control while walking. At this point, you may be able to wean off of the knee brace, but be sure to check with your surgeon or physical therapist first.

During the second week after ACL surgery, you will continue to focus on knee extension in various positions and work towards 90-100 degrees of knee flexion. Your physical therapist may add new exercises, like the ones below, to further develop your strength and knee control.

Mini squats

* Remove your knee brace. Stand behind a countertop or table and place both hands firmly on the surface. Position your feet about hip-width apart.

* Gently bend at the hips and knees, as if you are going to sit down on a high chair.

* Making sure your heels remain on the ground, pause for a few seconds before rising back to the starting position.

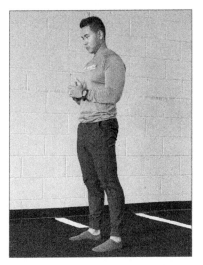 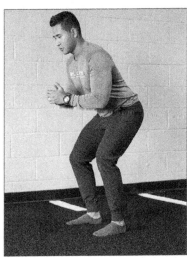

Figure 5: Mini-squat.

Heel raises (seated and standing)

✱ Stand behind a countertop or table and place both hands firmly on the surface. Position your feet about hip-width apart.

✱ Using your hands for stabilization, gently raise the heels off the floor and onto the balls of your feet.

✱ Hold for 5 seconds and ease slowly back down.

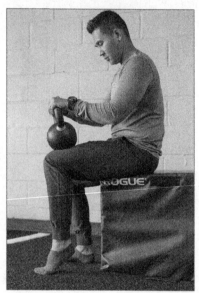 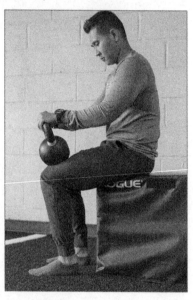

Figure 6: Sitting heel raises.

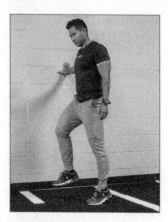

Figure 7: Standing heel raises.

Stationary bike

✱ Riding a stationary bike is encouraged once you can bend your knee at least 100 degrees.

✱ The seat position should be set to where the ball of the foot is in contact with the pedal with a slight bend at the knee when the pedal is closest to the ground.

✱ Use little-to-no resistance for the first few rides.

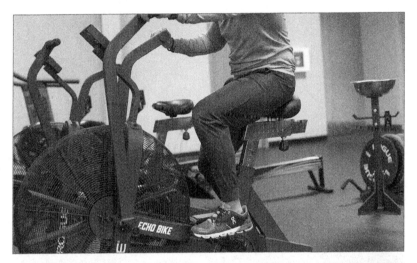

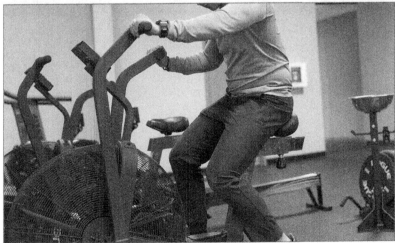

Figure 8: Biking forward/backward.

Side hip abduction

* Lie on your side with both legs straight. You should wear your knee brace for this exercise if you're unable to complete a straight leg raise.

* Keeping the toes pointed forward, raise the top leg about 10-12 inches towards the ceiling.

* Pause for a few seconds and slowly return to the starting position.

* Practice on both sides.

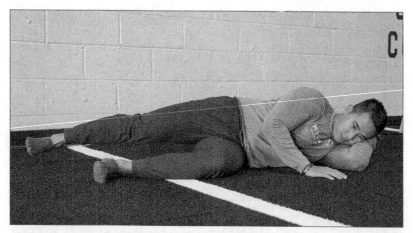

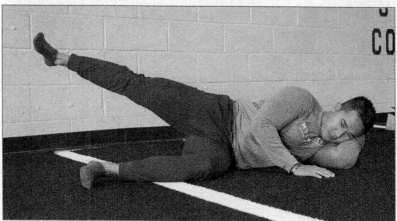

Figure 9: Side-lying hip abduction.

Bridging

* Lie on your back and bend both legs comfortably. Arms should rest at your sides.

* Squeeze the glutes as you lift your hips towards the ceiling.

* Pause at the top for 5 seconds and lower back to the starting position.

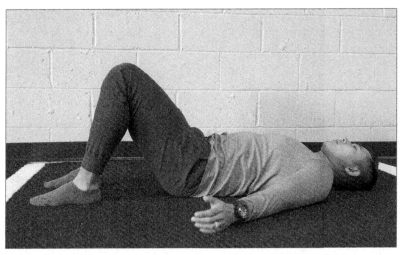

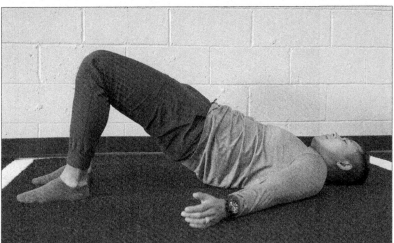

Figure 10: Bridges.

Modified deadlifts

* Standing with your feet about hip-width apart. Using light dumbbells or a kettlebell, hold firmly onto the weight.

* Keeping your back and legs straight, slowly lower the weight towards the ground. Push your hips back while keeping the heels on the ground.

* Stop when you've reached the middle of your shins.

* Squeeze your glutes as you push your hips forward to return to the starting position.

This book is accompanied by a catalog of exercises, as well as some additional information, which you can find by scanning the QR code below.

Criteria to Progress to Phase II

Remember, recovery happens at an individual pace, and it's difficult to predict recovery timeframes for everyone who suffers an ACL injury. However, there are a certain number of markers that suggest you're ready to move on from Phase I after ACL surgery.

Signs that you are ready to begin Phase II of ACL recovery and exercises are:

* Quad strength begins to return and you're able to do a straight leg raise without quad lag

* You can fully straighten your knee

* You are able to walk normally without crutches

* There's minimal-to-no knee swelling

Chapter 6

Phase II Rehab after ACL Surgery

A s you move forward with your recovery, things start to get a little more intense. The stage of recovery that usually begins in the third week after surgery and lasts until week 12 is known as Phase II.

Phase II is a big deal because it sets you up for success when it comes to making a full recovery. Because this phase is such a long part of the ACL rehabilitation process, it's best to split it up into three sections: Early, Mid, and Late Phase II.

Each portion of Phase II will have slightly different goals, but they are all connected to one another. Remember how we talked about short-term goals? This is where they become important.

This article will lay the groundwork for you to understand more about Phase II rehab after surgery for an ACL tear. First, we'll explain it all: your goals, exercises (also known as interventions), and criteria to move on. Then, we'll go into detail on how to perform the different exercises you'll be doing.

Let's jump right into the first section, Early Phase II.

This book is accompanied by a catalog of exercises, as well as some additional information, which you can find by scanning the QR code below.

Early Phase II

Your only goals during early phase II are to regain full extension of the operated knee, walk normally, and, most importantly, protect your newly-repaired ACL. Yes, these are all baby steps – but they're some of the most crucial ones you'll have. The good news is, it shouldn't take longer than a couple of weeks.

So, how do you achieve these goals? Do this by continuing to focus on range of motion, strength, and proprioception.

Continue to increase your knee range of motion.

Once you're able to bend your knee about 100 degrees, it's safe to try the stationary bike. This is a great way to keep working on your range of motion while beginning to get active again. Set the bike up so that the seat hits the top of your hip bone when you're standing next to it. Start slow and use gentle movements, especially when the pedals reach the 12 o'clock position.

Don't forget to do your daily stretches. The two stretches that are most beneficial to the early phase II goals of ACL recovery are:

Side-lying quad stretch – lying on the table, pull your heel to your glutes.

Standing quad stretch – standing on your unoperated leg, pull the heel of your operated leg to your glutes.

Continue with strengthening exercises, particularly those using your body weight.

The exercises you learned in Chapter 5 (Phase I) are still important in this phase. Continue working on your straight leg raises and hip strength. You can also try to incorporate some of the exercises below. As your strength improves, increase the weight as tolerated or instructed by your physical therapist.

✳ Hamstring curls

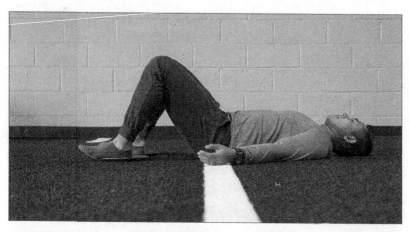

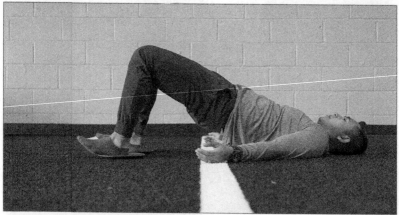

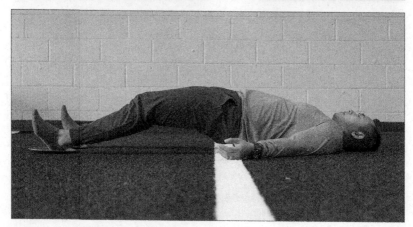

Figure 11: Hamstring curls.

* Step-ups

* Step-ups with marching

* Partial squats

* Goblet squats

* Kettlebell deadlift

* Ball squats and wall slides (to 60 degrees of knee flexion)

* Core strengthening

* Bridge

* One-legged bridge

* Bridge on an exercise ball

* Sideways hip clamshells

This book is accompanied by a catalog of exercises, as well as some additional information, which you can find by scanning the QR code below.

Introduce proprioception activities.

Proprioception is the body's awareness of where it is in space at any given moment. After ACL surgery, proprioception needs to be retrained because it's so crucial to lower body stability. This is done by challenging the body with different balancing exercises.

Single leg balance is the number one exercise when it comes to proprioception. Once you've mastered that, you can add unsteady surfaces to your routine. Whether it's a BOSU ball or a foam pad, unsteady surfaces increase the exercise's level of difficulty. Sideways stepovers should also be incorporated into the early phase of proprioception interventions.

Ok, so you did all of that. How do you know when you can move on to Mid-phase II of ACL recovery?

The criteria to progress includes:

✱ No swelling – especially not after your knee exercises.

✱ You should be able to bend your operated knee as much (or within 10 degrees) as the strong knee.

✱ You should be able to straighten the operated leg as much as the strong leg.

Check off all of those boxes, and you're ready for what's next.

Mid Phase II

Mid-phase II is where things get a little more intense. New phase, new goals.

Now that you've hit important milestones with your knee range of motion, it's time to make sure that you keep it. Along with that, you'll start to add onto your strengthening routine. Don't forget to watch your form and continue to protect the integrity of your new ACL.

You can expect to run through this portion of rehabilitation until you're about eight weeks out from ACL surgery.

No need to be repetitive, so don't worry about learning any new range of motion exercises during this phase. You're so close to being back to where you were before the ACL injury. Continue doing these exercises, along with the other interventions from Early Phase II, as you progress through Mid-phase II.

What To Expect for Cardiovascular Fitness During Mid Phase II Recovery from ACL Surgery

Although there's no new range of motion exercises, you do get to slowly reintroduce different forms of cardio. Hop on the stationary bike, elliptical, or stair climber to get your heart pumping. If you'd like to get in the pool, try out some light flutter kicks or pool jogging. However, hold off on land jogging for now.

What To Expect for Strengthening During Mid Phase II Recovery from ACL Surgery

We said it was time to increase the intensity, right? Well, we weren't kidding.

Say hello again to the gym. Using gym equipment is important during this time because it is an effective way to improve your quad and hamstring strength. You'll most likely use these machines:

* Leg press

* Box squat

* Barbell deadlift

* RDL

* Lunges

* Seated hamstring curl

* Hip abductor and adductor

* Hip extension

* Roman chair

* Seated calf

This book is accompanied by a catalog of exercises, as well as some additional information, which you can find by scanning the QR code below.

As always, make sure to follow the instructions on the machine for proper use. For your first time back on the machines, double-check your form with your physical therapist.

Some other exercises you can incorporate during this phase include squat to chair, lateral lunges, and Romanian deadlifts. Feel free to add handheld weights as you progress through the next few weeks.

At this point, you'll also begin a single leg strengthening progression. Once you've mastered one, your physical therapist will let you know when it's time to move on to the next. The progression goes as follows:

* Partial weight-bearing single leg press

* Single leg slide board lunges (reverse and lateral)

* Single leg step-ups (and with march)

* Lateral single-leg step-ups

* Single leg step downs

* Single leg squats

* Single leg wall slides

This book is accompanied by a catalog of exercises, as well as some additional information, which you can find by scanning the QR code below.

What To Expect for Proprioception During Mid Phase II Recovery from ACL Surgery

You'll do the same exercises from Early Phase II but add perturbations. This sounds complicated, but it's as easy as having someone tap different parts of your upper body while you're completing the exercises. This throws off your balance and trains your body to regain it.

Once you've hit all of your goals here, you can move onto Late Phase II. Just make sure that your range of motion matches your uninjured knee, and you're not experiencing pain or swelling when completing your exercises.

Late Phase II

Your goals are the same as Mid-Phase II, except this time, we turn it up a notch and add in training that's relevant to your sport, known as sport-specific movements. We'll utilize these interventions up to 12 weeks after your ACL surgery.

Though you obviously won't be ready to hit the field just yet, we can incorporate submaximal sport-specific movements in Late Phase II. This means low intensity, not full effort. All sport-specific movements should be forward, backward, upward, or downward motions. Skip the lateral or rotational exercises for now.

We can also introduce plyometrics, starting with partial weight-bearing exercises with both legs and progressing to full weight-bearing. No single leg plyometrics, like single-leg jumping, should be performed at this time.

Phase II Exercises

There were quite a few exercises for this part of your ACL recovery, and it's important to do them correctly. Here, we'll explain how to properly perform the interventions above.

Prone hamstring curls

* Attach your ankle weights to both legs.

* Lying on your stomach, bring the heel of your operated leg to your buttocks.

* Control the foot as you lower it back to the starting position.

Step ups

* Standing in front of a 6" step, place your operated leg onto the step.

* Shift your weight forward as you rise onto the step.

* Bring the uninjured leg onto the step.

* Slowly step down, one leg at a time, leading with your unoperated leg.

* Practice on both sides.

* To progress, add ankle weights or small handheld weights.

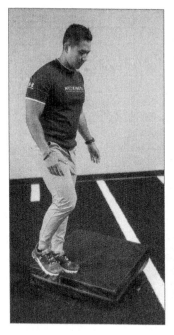 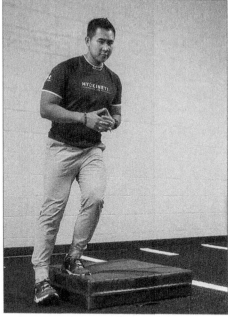

Figure 12: Step-up.

Step-ups with marching

* This exercise is performed similarly to the previous exercise.

* Instead of following with the unoperated leg, flex at the hip and bring the knee towards the ceiling as if you are marching.

* Lower the unoperated leg back to the ground and step down.

* Practice on both sides.

* To progress, add ankle weights.

Box squats

* With your feet hip-width apart, lower into a squat position while keeping your heels on the ground.

* Pause for a few seconds before standing. Think about driving your heels into the ground as you rise up.

* Bend to comfortable from 60-90 degrees until instructed to do so by your physical therapist.

* Use a kettlebell or a barbell.

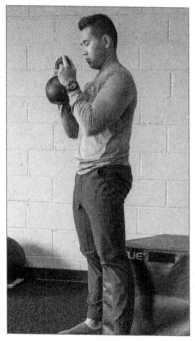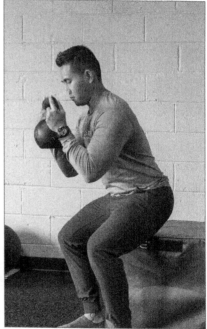

Figure 13: Box squat/Goblet squat.

Single leg squats

* Stand on one leg

* Contract your abdominals and slowly lower into a control range of motion squat.

* Pause and return back to a standing position.

* Avoid bending past 60 degrees until instructed to do so by your physical therapist.

Wall slides (Roman chair)

* Stand directly against a wall with your feet hip-width apart.

* Slowly slide down the wall until you reach a partial squat.

* Pause and rise back to a standing position.

* Avoid bending past 60 degrees until instructed to do so by your physical therapist.

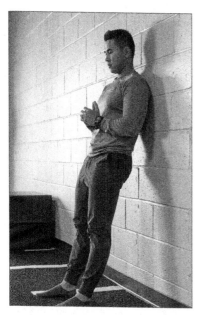
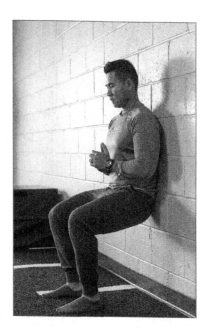

Figure 14: Wall sit.

Hip Thrust

✳ Lie on your back on a bench with your arms at your side and knees bent.

✳ Lift your hips off the ground until your body is in a straight line from your shoulders to your knees.

✳ Hold for 5 seconds by squeezing your glutes and slowly lower back down.

✳ Progress to single-leg bridges.

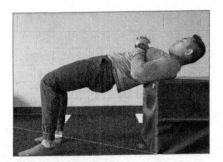 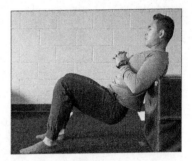

Figure 15: Hip thrust.

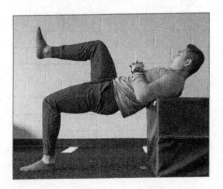 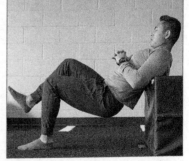

Figure 16: Single-leg hip thrust.

Bridge on an exercise ball

* Lie on your back with your arms at your side and knees bent. Place both feet on an exercise ball.

* Raise your hips towards the ceiling as you pull the ball towards your glutes with your heels.

* Straighten the legs as you slowly lower back down.

Sideways hip clamshells

* Lie on your side with both knees bent.

* Lift the top knee towards the ceiling while keeping your ankles together.

* Repeat on both sides.

* Increase the intensity of this exercise by wrapping a resistance band around your thighs.

Introduction to plyometrics

* Landing mechanics

* Jumping mechanics

* Jumping into landing

* Box jump

We gave you a ton of information to digest, so be sure to bookmark this for future reference. Once you achieve the goals in Phase II, you will be on your way to Phase III of ACL recovery.

The criteria to do so are:

* No signs of instability in the knee

* Maintain quad strength in both legs

* Good control and proper form when performing all range of motion, strengthening, and plyometric exercises

* Maintain balance on one leg for great than 30 seconds

Chapter 7

Phase III Rehab after ACL Surgery

At this stage, you're probably itching to get back to your normal routine, and rightly so. It's been a long 12+ weeks, but the end is in sight.

For the next two months, your ACL recovery will be focused on "the fun stuff." Things like sport-specific movements, agility, and plyometric activities will slowly be incorporated into your rehabilitation while still avoiding motions that cause pain. By now, you're probably good friends with your physical therapist and will continue to see him/her once or twice per week.

During Phase III for ACL recovery and rehabilitation, your primary goals are to strengthen and slowly reintroduce running, agility, and plyometric activities. This is done in a gradual manner and will require the expertise of your physical therapist. This chapter focuses on sharing ways in which these goals are achieved; more specifically, how to return to running after ACL surgery.

Before You Get Started

Before we discuss how to return to running after ACL surgery, it's important to understand that you must continue your strengthening and proprioceptive activities. Exercises like straight leg raises, partial squats, leg press, hamstring curls, and calf strengthening should be done on a regular basis. Work on increasing your strength and increase the weights as you're able.

You should also practice various balance exercises, like variations of single-leg balance, using balance boards, foam, and the BOSU ball. You can even begin outdoor biking, but only on flat roads. Hold off on mountain biking for now.

You may be wondering why you still need to do these things if you're getting stronger. It's because strengthening and balance exercises add protection to the knee joint and allow the ACL to continue to repair as you increase your activity level. Hip strengthening in particular becomes vital to prevent poor movement patterns while jumping or running. Core strength and stability of the lower body are useful to prevent rotation and maintain control while running.

So it should come as no surprise to you that you're going to need full knee range of motion, decent strength, and no signs of swelling before you begin any return-to-running program. Your surgeon and physical therapist may have other criteria such as a passing score on specific functional assessments, especially if you've also had a meniscus repair. Examples of functional tests include hopping forward, laterally, and/or light jogging.

And, before you lace up your running shoes, check with your surgeon to see if you need a functional sports brace. He or she may have a preference but, if not, your physical therapist will be able to offer more insight as to which knee brace will fit your needs.

This book is accompanied by a catalog of exercises, as well as some additional information, which you can find by scanning the QR code below.

ACL Return to Running Program

In a nutshell, here's the general progression of a return-to-running program after ACL surgery.

* Forward and backward jogging

* Jogging in different directions

* Speed and agility drills

Typically you'll begin with light intensity runs on soft surfaces for 3–4 days per week. It's recommended to start for 10 minutes at least for the first two weeks before gradually increasing your time given there's no pain or swelling in the knee joint. You'll want to avoid drastic fluctuations in mileage as this can lead to injury. Instead, follow the 10% rule: stay below a 10% increase in mileage per week.

But returning to running after ACL surgery involves more than monitoring your time and mileage. It's not unusual for your physical therapist to invest time working on your technique and running form during this phase. He or she will set parameters to help you avoid fatigue and encourage equal weight-bearing on both legs. You'll also learn how to land with your midfoot, as opposed to your heel, and improve your awareness of how your body moves.

Of equal importance is your ability to decelerate or accelerate. By learning how to decelerate properly, you'll be able to safely absorb forces to transition to your next movement, whether that is another step or a jump. Both of these skills need to be mastered before moving onto speed and agility, which trains your body to move in a different direction.

While you should keep in mind that each surgeon and physical therapist will have their own return-to-running protocols, here are examples of what you should expect.

Example of a Return-to-Jogging Protocol on the Treadmill

Day	1	2	3	4	5	6	7
Week 1	0.1 mile walk, 0.1 mile jog (10x total)	0.1 mile walk, 0.1 mile jog (10x total)			0.1 mile walk, 0.1 mile jog (10x total)		
Week 2				0.1 mile walk, 0.2 mile jog (2 miles)			0.1 mile walk, 0.2 mile jog (2 miles)
Week 3			0.1 mile walk, 0.3 mile jog (2 miles)			0.1 mile walk, 0.3 mile jog (2 miles)	
Week 4		0.1 mile walk, 0.4 mile jog (2 miles)		0.1 mile walk, 0.4 mile jog (2 miles)		2 mile jog	

Example of a Return to Running Protocol on the Treadmill

Day	1	2	3	4	5	6	7
Week 5		2 mile jog		2 mile jog		2 mile jog	
Week 6		2.5 mile jog		2.5 mile jog		3 mile jog	
Week 7	3 mile jog		3 mile jog		Alternate between run/jog every ¼ mile		
Week 8	Alternate between run/jog every ¼ mile		Alternate between run/jog every ¼ mile		Alternate between run/jog every ½ mile		Alternate between run/jog every ½ mile

ACL Return to Plyometrics: Jumping, Hopping, and Landing

Before you embark on this type of program, be sure to have full support from your surgeon and physical therapist. A return-to-plyometrics program after ACL surgery requires skilled expertise from a physical therapist and involves several different stages over a number of weeks.

Like the return-to-running program, you'll begin with low amplitude, low-velocity drills that work on your jumping and landing technique. During that time, you'll focus on something called landing mechanics which refers to your ability to bend at the hips, knees, and ankles to absorb force as you land. From there, you'll shift your attention to jumping mechanics to learn how to explode from the ground using your glutes, quads, and calf muscles.

Examples of low amplitude, low-velocity drills are forward and backward skipping, side shuffle, carioca, crossovers, backward jogging, shallow jump landings, and medicine ball squat catches. As you progress, your physical therapist will review proper ways to jump and land on one leg, especially when moving laterally.

Again, like the return-to-running protocol, your surgeon and physical therapist may have specific guidelines for you to follow. However, here's a general idea of what's to come during a return-to-plyometric program.

This book is accompanied by a catalog of exercises, as well as some additional information, which you can find by scanning the QR code below.

Phase 1: Forward and backward movements

* Shuttle press machine

* Box jumps

* Tuck jumps

* High knee

* ACDC

* Doubles

* Triples

* Bounding

* Deceleration drill

Phase 2: Lateral movements

* Side shuffle

* Carioca

* Shuttle run

* Zig-zag running

* Lateral ladder drills

Phase 3: Multidirectional movements

* Box drills

* Star drills

* Jump turns

* Box jumps with changes in direction

PHASE 4: SINGLE LEG PLYOMETRICS

* Single leg landing mechanics

* Jumping and landing

* Single leg hop

* Single leg triple hop

* Single leg crossover hop

* Single leg box jump

Criteria to Progress to Phase IV

Due to the intense sport-like demands of Phase IV of ACL recovery, you must meet the following milestones in order to move on. Here are the minimum requirements you'll need:

* Clearance from your surgeon and/or physical therapist

* Completion of the return-to-running program without pain or swelling in the knee joint

* Passing score on all functional assessments, like hopping on one leg

* Quad-to-hamstring ratio greater than 80%

* Quad-to-quad ratio greater than 90-95%

In addition to the physical criteria, you must demonstrate mental readiness on the Return to Sport after Injury (ACL RSI) scale. And, although you may pass the other tests with flying colors, it's possible that you're not mentally ready to go back on the field yet.

It's important to realize that you may harbor feelings of stress, anxiety, or fear about returning to the sport or activity that caused the injury. There is a possibility that, when left unaddressed, these feelings can evolve into fear-avoidance behaviors.

Fear-avoidance behaviors describe the way in which people avoid activities that they once enjoyed out of fear of a negative outcome. Furthermore, these behaviors are associated with poor performance despite being physically capable of doing well during practice or games. On the other hand, higher levels of self-confidence and low reports of fear are associated with better outcomes from ACL surgery. The possibility of you returning to your previous level of competition is higher than those with less confidence and greater reports of fear.

From mild apprehension or severe fear-avoidance behaviors, the psychological effects of returning to play should be addressed in everyone.[13] Therefore, don't be surprised if your physical therapist asks you to complete the ACL RSI scale during this phase.

---

13   Sibilski, C. (2021, April 8.) *How To Tell If Your Kid Is Ready to Play After an ACL Tear.* Myokinteix Physical Therapy and Performance. https://www. myokinetix.com/post/how-to-tell-if-your-kid-is-ready-to-play-after-an-acl-tear.

Chapter 8
Phase IV Rehab after ACL Surgery

Congratulations – you've made it to the end of your ACL rehab. Phase IV is the last stage before you officially get back on the field, and most would consider it to be the best part of the process. Not only is this stage full of sport-specific activities, but it's also a great confidence booster that will make you feel more at ease as you approach the end of your ACL recovery.

Before we dive into the events of Phase IV, take a moment to remember how far you've come. From a simple straight leg raise to a weight-based strengthening program to a running program; the past 20 weeks have prepared you for the upcoming sport-specific program. You've come a long way, and that's something to celebrate.

Some things to remember as you progress into Phase IV:

* Wear your knee brace – that's a no-brainer.

* Continue strengthening that knee – yes, you still need to do single-leg raises.

* Keep working on your balance – you're all too familiar with those single-leg balancing exercises by now.

* Maintain the Hamstring-to-quad ratio (around 70%) – no shock here, either.

Sport-Specific Movements

Whether you play football, hockey, soccer, or basketball, every sport has specific movements that define it. For soccer, those movements are kicking, cutting, dribbling, and dodging defenders. In volleyball, sport-specific movements include planting and jumping, leaping, and serving. The most crucial part of Phase IV of ACL recovery is finding a way to incorporate those aspects of your sport into your ACL rehab.

Fortunately, there is a safe way to do this while avoiding injury to the healing ACL reconstruction. To help you understand these concepts, we'll use soccer as an example.

If you successfully completed your running program and achieved other criteria in Phase III, then you're cleared to do more complex plyometric and agility drills during Phase IV. As with all other phases of ACL rehab, reintroduction to soccer plyometrics and agility drills begins incrementally with low-intensity drills. For example, use a soccer ball to slowly work on your touches and passing skills. Once you're comfortable with that, progress to shooting drills and dribbling laterally with light cutting.

Your plyometric exercises should be sport-specific as well. Add a passing drill or a dribbling exercise to multidirectional jumps. You can also practice catching balls thrown by your coach or athletic trainer after jumping on top of a plyometric box (this one is particularly fun for a goalkeeper).

ACL Return to Practice

Non-contact drills play a big part in the progression of Phase IV ACL rehab. Once you've gained some confidence from your sport-specific agility and plyometrics activities, you can enter into non-contact drills at practice. The definition of non-contact can vary from sport to sport, but it typically means that you should avoid contact with a teammate, the ground, or objects.

When it comes time to participate in full-contact drills at practice, do so lightly and slowly ease your way into it. Rushing back into a full-contact practice like you never left is extremely dangerous and places you at high risk for ACL re-injury, which is something you definitely want to avoid.

Once you can safely participate in a full practice, celebrate this milestone. This is a huge part of what you've been working toward. The next step is your final goal – to play in a full game.

ACL Return To Play

Just like with every other exercise or drill you've encountered throughout your ACL rehab, returning to play after ACL surgery should be done gradually. Just because you've been able to complete a full practice without restrictions doesn't mean you can play all 60 minutes during the next soccer game.

Because game situations can't always be simulated in practice, start with a scrimmage with your teammates. For your first scrimmage, play for 10 minutes in each half. This is a safe starting point from a physical and mental standpoint. Increase your time on the field with each scrimmage played so long as you don't experience any discomfort along the way.

When it comes time to play a refereed game, use a sliding scale based upon percentage of total playing time. Begin with 5-10% per half/period/quarter and increase based upon your medical providers' recommendations. Keep in mind that you're going against athletes on the opposing team, which heightens the intensity (and risk) of game situations.

The most important thing to do in this stage is to advocate for yourself. If you don't feel right, tell a coach, teammate, or your trainer. Find the courage to pull yourself from the scrimmage (or the game) if something feels off. Keeping pain or discomfort to yourself is detrimental and will hinder you from getting back to 100%.

Continued Monitoring

Now that you're more active, it's likely that your knee will be tired at the end of practice. That is usually a good sign since it means you're getting stronger and steadier on your feet. However, watch out for swelling and pain since those are signs that indicate you overdid it.

You should be feeling pretty confident about where you're at now. Don't forget to check in with your physical therapist throughout this phase of your rehab. Although you're back at practice and not in one-on-one treatment sessions with your PT, you should be touching base every 2 weeks or so as you progress.

Remember – you're not going to be in the same shape as you were prior to your ACL surgery. Don't let this discourage you, though. Give yourself grace as you recondition your body to return to your peak athletic shape. As stated earlier, you've come a long way, and this is the home stretch.

Once you've completed a full game, you have achieved every goal and milestone of your ACL recovery, and there are no additional criteria to move on. It's been a long nine months, but you did it. You have reached the finish line, and you deserve to celebrate that win. Well done!

Chapter 9

Lifelong Management of ACL Injuries

Now that you have completed the return-to-play process after ACL surgery, it's time to talk about life after recovery from an ACL tear.

Should you be concerned about a possible reinjury? Are you at risk for early onset of arthritis? What type of things can be done to prevent those conditions? It's natural to have these questions, and others, as you start attending practice regularly.

While we explored ACL reinjury rate earlier in the series, let's take some time to delve into early onset arthritis and other challenges you may face after ACL recovery. Then, we will discuss the importance of lifetime management and how to keep your ACL reconstruction healthy in the years to come.

Role of Physical Therapy During ACL Recovery

It's a well-known fact that physical therapy after an ACL injury is as critical as the surgery itself when it comes to getting back to sports and exercise. Physical therapy is also a large part of whether ACL surgery is considered to be successful, and that's because it sets the stage for what you're able to do for the rest of your life.

For people who are looking to return to sports and exercise, physical therapy after an ACL injury is necessary to help you regain range of motion, strength, speed, and agility. But what happens when they don't complete enough?

There is a significantly increased risk of reinjury to the ACL that had previously been injured, as well as a risk of tearing the opposite ACL due to asymmetry and muscle imbalance taxing the nonsurgical knee to a greater extent.

Research suggests that athletes do not return to the same level of competition for up to 2 years after ACL surgery. This is one of the reasons why ACL return-to-play testing is highly encouraged. Generally, return-to-play testing after ACL surgery includes a strength evaluation, functional activities like hopping, jump/landing, and sports-specific activities. Once you pass the return-to-play milestone, research shows that you have a good prognosis for playing at the same level you did prior to the injury.

On the other hand, some milestones, like regaining full range of motion or strength, during ACL recovery may be difficult to meet. Although there are many factors that can affect overall recovery, some can place you at risk for poorer outcomes. People who fail to regain full knee range of motion, the recommended quad-to-hamstring ratio, and normal jumping/landing patterns are more susceptible to developing arthritis. Afterwards, the knee joint can develop chronic inflammation that results in changes to the joint structure and damage to the cartilage.

Why ACL Recovery Occurs Over a Lifetime

We make this claim for two reasons, so hear us out.

Firstly, it takes about two years for your nervous system to reconnect with your balance and proprioceptive systems after an ACL injury. During this time, you are extremely vulnerable to ACL reinjury; a fact that highlights the importance of periodic check-ins with your physical therapist or trainer.

Secondly, about one third of people who undergo ACL surgery will develop osteoarthritis in the injured knee within 10 years. Within two decades, nearly 50 percent will have osteoarthritis which emphasizes a strong need for better education and prevention programs for those who are at risk.

Arthritis after ACL injury, also known as post-traumatic osteoarthritis (PTOA), is a subtype of osteoarthritis that develops after an injury to the joint such as a fracture or a ligament/meniscus injury. It accounts for almost 12% of arthritis cases and disproportionately affects younger populations due to a higher percentage of the traumatic injuries that cause PTOA. Other conditions that can lead to PTOA include shoulder instability, patellar dislocation, and ankle instability.

There are certain defining features of PTOA during the early stages. While there is no definitive cure for PTOA, or osteoarthritis, this means that targeted treatments could potentially prevent the disease from progressing and causing symptoms.

Currently, there is strong research in support of there being help for those with symptomatic PTOA. Experts recommend making healthy lifestyle choices, like quitting smoking and eating well, to prevent symptoms related to PTOA. Furthermore, developing realistic expectations and finding ways to control flare-ups is helpful to manage PTOA. Things like anti-inflammatory diets, routinely engaging in physical activity, and consuming nutrients for bone health (calcium, vitamin D, and omega-3 fatty acids) are also recommended to combat the effects and progression of PTOA.

Unsurprisingly, though, the most effective way to manage PTOA is prevention of injury and reinjury. ACL prevention programs play a large role in protecting the ligaments, meniscus, and knee joint and can reduce the rate of injury by up to 53%. These programs should include neuromuscular and proprioceptive training, strengthening, plyometrics, balance, and flexibility exercises along with feedback on technique and skill enhancement. Altogether, ACL prevention programs improve lower body mechanics and offer greater protection against future ACL injury.

One example of a well-known ACL prevention program, the FIFA 11+, was developed in 2006 as a warm-up routine aimed at preventing soccer injuries in individuals ages 13 years old and up. One study found that FIFA 11+ decreased the rate of ACL injuries by 77%, an impressive statistic for such a highly competitive contact sport. Although FIFA 11+ was originally designed for soccer, the idea can be easily put to use in other sports with high ACL injury rates.

Chapter 10

Why Myokinetix Is Your #1 Resource for ACL Injury

We've just shown you what ACL rehabilitation looks like and how you, your surgeon, and your physical therapist all play significant roles in your ACL injury treatment.

For the best chance of a smooth recovery, find a physical therapist who:

* Specializes in ACL rehabilitation.

* Understands your sport and position – this will help you set those short-term goals.

* Is familiar with your particular sport or activity.

* Works in an environment that works for you. Athletes benefit from settings that make them feel like an athlete. Adequate equipment and the state of the facility are key factors in the recovery environment.

ACL recovery should be considered a lifetime process due to the high rate of reinjury and risk for developing post-traumatic osteoarthritis. Therefore, it makes sense to put your recovery in the capable hands of a team who knows ACL rehabilitation from firsthand experience.

The doctors of physical therapy at Myokinetix value the importance of physical, mental, and emotional readiness, which is one of the reasons why you should trust their expertise in ACL recovery and rehabilitation. Their goals are to help you create a positive relationship with your body and motivate you throughout your ACL recovery. Let their experts become your #1 resource for ACL injury and recovery.

**Learn more about the Myokinetix ACL Rehab system
by calling +1 (973) 585-4990 today
or contact us at info@myokinetix.com
and work with us from anywhere in the world.**

www.myokinetix.com

References

Evans J, Nielson Jl. Anterior Cruciate Ligament Knee Injuries. [Updated 2021 Feb 19]. In: StatPearls [Internet]. Treasure Island (FL): StatPearls Publishing; 2021 Jan-. Available from: https://www.ncbi.nlm.nih.gov/books/NBK499848/

Shelbourne, K. & Benner, Rodney & Gray, Tinker. (2017). Results of Anterior Cruciate Ligament Reconstruction With Patellar Tendon Autografts: Objective Factors Associated With the Development of Osteoarthritis at 20 to 33 Years After Surgery. *The American Journal of Sports Medicine*. 45. 10.1177/0363546517718827.

Kane, Patrick & Wascher, Jocelyn & Dodson, Christopher & Hammoud, Sommer & Cohen, Steven & Ciccotti, Michael. (2016). Anterior cruciate ligament reconstruction with bone-patellar tendon-bone autograft versus allograft in skeletally mature patients aged 25 years or younger. *Knee Surgery, Sports Traumatology, Arthroscopy*. 24. 10.1007/s00167-016-4213-z.

Maletis, Gregory & Chen, Jason & Inacio, Maria & Love, Rebecca & Funahashi, Tadashi. (2017). Increased Risk of Revision After Anterior Cruciate Ligament Reconstruction With Bone–Patellar Tendon–Bone Allografts Compared With Autografts. *The American Journal of Sports Medicine*. 45. 036354651769038. 10.1177/0363546517690386.

Beischer, S., Gustavsson, L., Senorski, E. H., Karlsson, J., Thomeé, C., Samuelsson, K., & Thomeé, R. (2020). Young Athletes Who Return to Sport Before 9 Months After Anterior Cruciate Ligament Reconstruction Have a Rate of New Injury 7 Times That of Those

Who Delay Return. *Journal of Orthopaedic & Sports Physical Therapy,* 50(2), 83–90. doi: 10.2519/jospt.2020.9071

Gans, I., Retzky, J. S., Jones, L. C., & Tanaka, M. J. (2018). Epidemiology of Recurrent Anterior Cruciate Ligament Injuries in National Collegiate Athletic Association Sports: The Injury Surveillance Program, 2004-2014. *Orthopaedic Journal of Sports Medicine,* 6(6), 232596711877782. doi: 10.1177/2325967118777823

Joseph, A. M., Collins, C. L., Henke, N. M., Yard, E. E., Fields, S. K., & Comstock, R. D. (2013). A Multisport Epidemiologic Comparison of Anterior Cruciate Ligament Injuries in High School Athletics. *Journal of Athletic Training,* 48(6), 810–817. doi: 10.4085/1062-6050-48.6.03

Joseph AM, Collins CL, Henke NM, Yard EE, Fields SK, Comstock RD. A multisport epidemiologic comparison of anterior cruciate ligament injuries in high school athletics. *Journal of Athletic Training.* 2013;48(6):810-817. doi:10.4085/1062-6050-48.6.03

Gornitzky AL, Lott A, Yellin JL, Fabricant PD, Lawrence JT, Ganley TJ. Sport-Specific Yearly Risk and Incidence of Anterior Cruciate Ligament Tears in High School Athletes: A Systematic Review and Meta-analysis. *Am J Sports Med.* 2016;44(10):2716-2723. doi:10.1177/0363546515617742

American Academy of Orthopedic Surgeons website, Ortho Info. Anterior Cruciate Ligament (ACL) Injuries. Accessed May 16 2021.

Perrone GS, Proffen BL, Kiapour AM, Sieker JT, Fleming BC, Murray MM. Bench-to-bedside: Bridge-enhanced anterior cruciate ligament repair. *J Orthop Res.* 2017 Dec;35(12):2606-2612. doi: 10.1002/jor.23632. Epub 2017 Jul 9. Review. *PubMed PMID:* 28608618; PubMed Central PMCID: PMC5729057.

McGuine TA, Post EG, Hetzel SJ, Brooks MA, Trigsted S, Bell DR. A Prospective Study on the Effect of Sport Specialization on Lower Extremity Injury Rates in High School Athletes. *The American Journal of Sports Medicine.* 2017;45(12):2706-2712. doi:10.1177/0363546517710213

MOON Knee Group, Spindler, K. P., Huston, L. J., Chagin, K. M., Kattan, M. W., Reinke, E. K., Amendola, A., Andrish, J. T., Brophy, R. H., Cox, C. L., Dunn, W. R., Flanigan, D. C., Jones, M. H., Kaeding, C. C., Magnussen, R. A., Marx, R. G., Matava, M. J., McCarty, E. C., Parker, R. D., Pedroza, A. D., … Wright, R. W. (2018). Ten-Year Outcomes and Risk Factors After Anterior Cruciate Ligament Reconstruction: A MOON Longitudinal Prospective Cohort Study. *The American journal of sports medicine*, 46(4), 815–825. https://doi.org/10.1177/0363546517749850

Watt, F. E., Corp, N., Kingsbury, S. R., Frobell, R., Englund, M., Felson, D. T., Levesque, M., Majumdar, S., Wilson, C., Beard, D. J., Lohmander, L. S., Kraus, V. B., Roemer, F., Conaghan, P. G., Mason, D. J., & Arthritis Research UK Osteoarthritis and Crystal Disease Clinical Study Group Expert Working Group (2019). Towards prevention of post-traumatic osteoarthritis: report from an international expert working group on considerations for the design and conduct of interventional studies following acute knee injury. *Osteoarthritis and cartilage*, 27(1), 23–33. https://doi.org/10.1016/j.joca.2018.08.001

Wang, LJ., Zeng, N., Yan, ZP. et al. Post-traumatic osteoarthritis following ACL injury. *Arthritis Res Ther 22*, 57 (2020). https://doi.org/10.1186/s13075-020-02156-5

Brigham Young University. (2018, September 18). Long-term success of ACL reconstruction is connected to the way you move post-surgery: Study helps shed light on why so many ACL patients end up with osteoarthritis in the knee. *ScienceDaily*. Retrieved June 11, 2021 from www.sciencedaily.com/releases/2018/09/180918082043.htm

https://www.massgeneral.org/assets/MGH/pdf/orthopaedics/sports-medicine/physical-therapy/rehabilitation-protocol-for-ACL.pdf

https://www.sportsmednorth.com/sites/sportsmednorthV2/files/ACL-Reconstruction-Protocol.pdf

https://www.uwhealth.org/files/uwhealth/docs/sportsmed/ACL_Adult_Rehab.pdf

https://www.bostonsportsmedicine.com/pdf/protocols/acl_reconstruction_rehab_protocol.pdf

Sadeqi, M., Klouche, S., Bohu, Y., Herman, S., Lefevre, N., & Gerometta, A. (2018). Progression of the Psychological ACL-RSI Score and Return to Sport After Anterior Cruciate Ligament Reconstruction: A Prospective 2-Year Follow-up Study From the French Prospective Anterior Cruciate Ligament Reconstruction Cohort Study (FAST). *Orthopaedic journal of sports medicine, 6*(12), 2325967118812819. https://doi.org/10.1177/2325967118812819

Burland, J. P., Toonstra, J., Werner, J. L., Mattacola, C. G., Howell, D. M., & Howard, J. S. (2018). Decision to Return to Sport After Anterior Cruciate Ligament Reconstruction, Part I: A Qualitative Investigation of Psychosocial Factors. *Journal of Athletic Training (Allen Press), 53*(5), 452–463. https://doi.org/10.4085/1062-6050-313-16

Heijne, A., Axelsson, K., Werner, S., & Biguet, G. (2008). Rehabilitation and recovery after anterior cruciate ligament reconstruction: patients' experiences. *Scandinavian Journal of Medicine & Science in Sports, 18*(3), 325–335. https://doi.org/10.1111/j.1600-0838.2007.00700.x

K;, S. G. S. B. B. (2019, August). Rehabilitation and nutrition protocols for optimising return to play from traditional ACL reconstruction in elite rugby union players: A case study. *Journal of sports sciences.* https://pubmed.ncbi.nlm.nih.gov/30967011/

Mohammed, W. A., Pappous, A., & Sharma, D. (2018, May 15). Effect of Mindfulness Based Stress Reduction (MBSR) in Increasing Pain Tolerance and Improving the Mental Health of Injured Athletes. *Frontiers in psychology.* https://www.ncbi.nlm.nih.gov/pmc/articles/PMC5963333/

Petrie, K., & Matzkin, E. (2019). Can pharmacological and non-pharmacological sleep aids reduce post-operative pain and opioid usage? A review of the literature. *Orthopedic reviews, 11*(4), 8306. https://doi.org/10.4081/or.2019.8306

Rodriguez, T. (2013, May 1). Mental Imagery May Hasten Recovery after Surgery. *Scientific American*. https://www.scientificamerican.com/article/mental-imagery-may-hasten-recovery-after-surgery/

Tompkins, Marc, Plante, Matthew, Monchik, Keith, Fleming, Braden, & Fadale, Paul. (2011). The use of a non-benzodiazepine hypnotic sleep-aid (Zolpidem) in patients undergoing ACL reconstruction: A randomized controlled clinical trial. *Knee Surgery, Sports Traumatology, Arthroscopy : Official Journal of the ESSKA*, 19(5), 787-791.

Wiggins AJ, Grandhi RK, Schneider DK, Stanfield D, Webster KE, Myer GD. Risk of Secondary Injury in Younger Athletes After Anterior Cruciate Ligament Reconstruction: A Systematic Review and Meta-analysis. *Am J Sports Med*. 2016;44(7):1861-1876. doi:10.1177/0363546515621554

Howard M, Solaru S, Kang HP, et al. Epidemiology of Anterior Cruciate Ligament Injury on Natural Grass Versus Artificial Turf in Soccer. 10-Year Data From the National Collegiate Athletic Association Injury Surveillance System. *Orthop J Sports Med*. 2020;8(7):2325967120934434. Published 2020 Jul 22. doi:10.1177/2325967120934434

Beischer S, Gustavsson L, Senorski EH, et al. Young Athletes Who Return to Sport Before 9 Months After Anterior Cruciate Ligament Reconstruction Have a Rate of New Injury 7 Times That of Those Who Delay Return [published correction appears in *J Orthop Sports Phys Ther*. 2020 Jul;50(7):411]. *J Orthop Sports Phys Ther*. 2020;50(2):83-90. doi:10.2519/jospt.2020.9071

Nyman E Jr, Armstrong CW. Real-time feedback during drop landing training improves subsequent frontal and sagittal plane knee kinematics. *Clin Biomech (Bristol, Avon)*. 2015;30(9):988-994. doi:10.1016/j.clinbiomech.2015.06.018

Tipton KD. Nutritional Support for Exercise-Induced Injuries. *Sports Med*. 2015;45 Suppl 1:S93-S104. doi:10.1007/s40279-015-0398-4

Kehlet H. Enhanced postoperative recovery: good from afar, but far from good?. *Anaesthesia*. 2020;75 Suppl 1:e54-e61. doi:10.1111/anae.14860

Barber-Westin S, Noyes FR. One in 5 Athletes Sustain Reinjury Upon Return to High-Risk Sports After ACL Reconstruction: A Systematic Review in 1239 Athletes Younger Than 20 Years. *Sports Health.* *2020;*12(6):587-597. doi:10.1177/1941738120912846

Hilton L, Hempel S, Ewing BA, et al. Mindfulness Meditation for Chronic Pain: Systematic Review and Meta-analysis. *Ann Behav Med.* *2017;*51(2):199-213. doi:10.1007/s12160-016-9844-2

Printed in Great Britain
by Amazon

82887193R00058